CW00468455

Edizioni R.E.I. France

All our ebooks can be read on the following devices: computers, eReaders, IOS, android, blackberry, windows, tablets, mobile phones.

French Academy

The system of the seven Chakras (3)

Manipura - The third Chakra

ISBN 978-2-37297-3564

Edizioni R.E.I. France
www.edizionirei.webnode.com
edizionireifrance@outlook.com

French Academy

Manipura

The Third Chakra

Edizioni R.E.I. France

Index

The Chakra system

With the word Chakra, which derives from Sanskrit and means "wheel", we want to indicate the seven basic centers of energy in the human body. The chakras are centers of subtle psychic energy located along the spine. Each of these centers is connected, at the level of subtle energies, to the main ganglia of the nerves that branch out from the vertebral column. In addition, the chakras are related to the levels of consciousness, to the archetypal elements, to the phases inherent in the development of life, to colors, which are closely related to the Chakras, because they are located outside of our body, but within the aura, that is to say the electromagnetic field that surrounds each person, to the sounds, to the functions of the body and to much, much more. The Eastern doctrine that has spread knowledge in the Western world considers the Chakras as openings, access doors to the essence of the human body.

Chakras are usually represented inside a lotus flower, with a variable number of open petals. The open petals represent the chakra in its full opening. On each petal is written one of the fifty letters of the Sanskrit alphabet, which are considered sacred letters, then divine expression. Each of them also expresses a different activity of the human being, a different state of his, both manifest and still potential. Each chakra resonates on a different

9

frequency that corresponds to the colors of the rainbow.

The seven main Chakras also correspond to the seven main glands of our endocrine system. Their main function is to absorb the Universal Energy, to metabolize it, to break it down and to channel it along the energy channels up to the nervous system, to nourish the auras and release energy outside. Almost everyone sees them as funnels, which spin and simultaneously run the energy back and forth. Each of the seven centers has both a (usually dominant) front component and a (usually less dominant) rear component, which are intimately connected, except for the first and seventh, which are single. from the second to the fifth, the anterior aspect relates to the feelings and the emotions, while the posterior aspect with the will. Regarding the anterior and posterior sixth, and the seventh, the correlation is with mind and reason. The first and seventh. they also have the very important function of connection for the human being: being the outermost Chakras of the energetic channel, they have the characteristic of relating man with the Universe on one side and with the Earth on the other.

The perfect functioning of the energy system is synonymous with good health. To open the Chakras there are many different techniques, among which the Reiki stands out for its peculiar sweetness and for the possibility of harmonizing any energy imbalances. Each center oversees certain organs, and has particular functions on an emotional, psychic and spiritual level. Among the fundamental sects, precise affinities exist :

- First with Seventh: Basic Energy with Spiritual Energy.
- Second with Sesto: Energy of feeling on a material level with Energy of feeling on an extrasensory level.
- Third with Quintus: Energy of the operative mind and of personal power with Energy of the higher mind and of communication.
- Fourth: bridge between the three upper and the three lower and alchemical forge of transformation.

A color is associated with each Chakra, which corresponds and derives from the frequency and the vibration of the center itself. In addition to each Chakra corresponds a mantra, the sound of a musical note and, in some cases, also a natural element, a planet or a zodiacal sign. Because the chakra system is the primary processing center for every function of our being, the blockage or energetic insufficiency in the chakras usually causes disorders in the body, mind or spirit.

A defect in the flow of energy that passes through the given chakra will cause a defect in the energy supplied to the connected parts of the physical body, as it will affect all levels of being.

This is because an energy field is a holistic entity; every part of it affects every other part. Essential oils are able to tune into specific chakras: their scent and vibration gently bring us into deep contact with our energy centers.

The massage with specific essential oils on the points corresponding to the chakras, activates and balances their action, harmonizing and strengthening the whole organism.

Starting from the bottom are:

- 1st = Muladhara
- 2nd = Swadhisthana
- 3rd = Manipura
- 4th = Anahata
- 5th = Vhishuddhi
- 6th = Ajna
- 7th = Sahasrara

Moreover, each of the seven chakras comes to represent an important area of human psychic health, which we can briefly summarize as:

- 1 survival
- 2 sexuality
- 3 force
- 4 love
- 5 communication
- 6 intuition
- 7 cognition.

Metaphorically the chakras are related to the following archetypal elements:

- 1 land
- 2 water
- 3 fire

- 4 air
- 5 sound
- 6 light
- 7 thoughts.

Manipura - Third Chakra

The third chakra is called the solar plexus chakra, or the navel chakra. In Sanskrit language it is called Manipura, which means city of jewels.

It has as its symbol a yellow lotus flower with ten petals, on which are the letters Dam, Dham, Nam, Tam, Tham, Dam, Dham, Nam, Pam, Pham. At the center of the flower are the red triangle of Fire (Tejas), the syllable/root "Ram" and a ram, traditional messenger of Agni, the Hindu Lord of Fire. It is placed in the solar plexus/dome of the diaphragm.

From the psycho-energetic point of view, its most important function is related to the personal affirmation and the exercise of individual power with respect to the social and the environment in general; it indicates the realization of the person, how much the person sees his desire for life achievable, how much a person wants and wants to fight for himself, how much a person loves himself. It develops from 4/6 years until the end of childhood, around 10/12 years, allowing the boy/girl to gain independence and realize emotional separation from parents.

The main pathologies expressed by the third Chakra concern all metabolic diseases, such as diabetes, hyperlipidaemia, liver failure, cirrhosis, gastric and duodenal ulcers, glucose levels, and all pathologies concerning the processes of nutrition, digestion and assimilation.

From the psycho-energetic point of view it is at the level of this Chakra that the emotional forces directed towards the external environment are generated: the feelings of friendship, resentment, sympathy, antipathy.

The third chakra, in particular, is the expression of the awareness that each has of himself: that ability to feel pleasure in knowing how satisfied, but also the humility that distinguishes the one who knows he can always improve, because growth resides in change.

It is the Chakra of individual will, charisma and efficiency.

It is the foundation of the social personality.

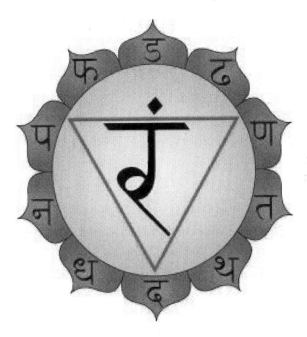

Excessive functioning causes incapacity to remain calm, outbursts of anger, hyperactivity, stomach disorders of nervous origin; the lacking functioning, on the other hand, causes little energy, shyness, continuous need to resort to exciters or stimulants.

The disharmonic functioning of this Chakra generates the unbridled desire of power, of manipulation, in order to overturn reality always and in its favor; tendentially we can notice a hyperactive attitude, which is put in place to hide the sense of inadequacy and emptiness that is caused by the impotence to manage the situations of absolute power that one would expect to exercise.

The inner serenity will be strongly compromised and, obviously, the satisfaction of material wellbeing will be the main one, even at the expense of any pleasant feeling, even coming to consider them undesirable and annoying.

The subject who suffers from a decompensation of the third Chakra is led to lose control of his emotions and develop a strongly aggressive attitude, necessary not to allow others to strip their inner weakness, this would unmask the power games of to whom this subject lives, creating a situation of energetic paralysis that would express itself as desperate and desperate impotence. An example of this defeated subject can be given by the image of those generally middle-aged people, but increasingly young people, who spend their time in annihilating and destructive activities, such as drinking, using drugs more or less less recognized as such, and generally have a strongly aggressive and overbearing attitude in the family.

In fact, these are followed by a highly depressive situation.

In this case the subject will have as main objective the being accepted and welcomed by others, and to achieve this purpose he will deny himself to conform to the way of thinking of the people he wishes to please, suffocating and completely denying his own desires and emotions; nevertheless, on the contrary, precisely because of this frustrating attitude, the arrogance and harassment of members of one's family will increase. Powerful and solar chakra, reveals to everyone their right to exist and their place in the Universe, promoting self-acceptance.

Through its totally harmonic expression, the human being is in the world with the fullness of his physical and mental attributes and allows him to act on the material plane in a loose and harmonious way, promoting the enjoyment of everything. If the third chakra is not perfectly harmonious it can nourish one's sense of inferiority; they can diminish their real mental abilities, such as logic and rationality, and increase, therefore, confusion and a sense of insecurity. It may happen that it feeds its own desire for power, possession and, consequently, even overpowering others to obtain and excel. Will and power represent for everyone, in the current society (especially Western), one of the keys to success, but can represent, when understood in an egoic sense of possession and hoarding, the impossibility of conscious access to the other chakras and, therefore, to a real fullness of one's own Being.

This center is also called Nabhi and is located in the solar plexus region just below the diaphragm. It is associated with individual and collective well-being, with the acceptance of one's neighbor, with individual willpower.

It would be linked to the stomach, intestine, liver, gallbladder, spleen, pancreas.

It would stop because of great scares (with stomach contraction) or because of reaction to situations or people that are not accepted and this block would cause incapacity to remain calm, outbursts of anger, hyperactivity, disorders of nervous origin. The element of this chakra is fire. .

The organ of sense related to the manipura are the eyes, seat of sight, while the organ of action is the anus, ie the excretory apparatus (however also connected with muladhara) which conveys downwards the slags produced by the process of transformation and assimilation that the fire performs. The main characteristic of this chakra is the heat for which the concentration operated on it favors heating and combustion. The bijamantra is "ram", ie the nasalized "ra" letter. It is the bijamantra of the god Agni, lord of the fire mounted on the ram, visualized as a divinity by the color of the rising sun, flaming, with four arms that hold in two hands the rosary and the lance, while the other two are posed in the gesture that dissipates fear and in the gesture of the gift. In the dot that is placed on the letter to nasalize it is inscribed another deity, Rudra, or the god Shiva, the dissolver of the universe, here represented as an old vermilion incarnato, sprinkled with ashes, with three eyes and two arms, the hands posed in the gesture that dispels fear and bestows gifts, sitting on the bull Nandin, his mount.

The Shakti here is projected as Lakini, terrifying goddess on a red lotus, drunken ambrosia, flamboyant, dark blue, dressed in yellow, with fangs, three faces with a third eye in each, four arms, with the lance and the thunderbolt in two hands and the other two in the gesture that dissipates fear and in that of the gift. It is delicious with meat and is associated with muscle tissue.

The energy of the chakra is further specified by the presence within the triangle of a ram, also a symbol of solar power, of the power of fire, of an active energy, and of two gods, Rudra and Lakini: the first is the transformer of creation, the second the benefactor. The one separates, the other reunites allowing all things to enter into a relationship with each other. On the other hand, the planet that the ancient esoteric schools make correspond to this chakra is Mercury, because it is precisely the symbol of the ability to connect, to relate things to each other: the winged Mercury, suspended between earth and sky.

In the area where this chakra is located there is a very important plexus of the SNA, the solar plexus which represents the focal point of the innervation of the digestive system: the digestive function is in fact entirely "controlled" by this plexus through the action of two "hollow" organs, the stomach and the intestine, and of two important "full" organs, the liver and pancreas.

Another small hollow organ is linked to the liver: the gall bladder. These organs allow digestion and assimilation of food; this means that food, part of the extra-individual world that is brought into the individual, arrives in the stomach, biological "furnace" where, through a chemical fire (for example hydrochloric acid), food is digested, "burned" », Ie its form and individuality is destroyed, it is transformed into its simplest components, also through the action of the liver and pancreas, in such a way as to pass into the intestine, a place where food, by now transformed, is assimilated , that is, brought into the blood, in direct contact with the individual who ate it, and then became part of its own cells, that is, its integral part. In this way the individual and extra-individual world come into contact, they transform each other. Therefore we are told "we are what we eat", because that particular type of "energy" that we introduce remains within us, becomes part of us and, as a part that belongs to us, we can also know it (or "recognize it"?).

The digestive system therefore has the function of relating the individual to the external world through a separating and destructive fire, which then allows an assimilation, that is a beneficial meeting within a single individuality. . We note here that the prerogative of man to be, unique among all animals, omnivorous, that is to be able to feed on any food, places it once again at the apex of evolution. In fact, if we continue in this interpretation of the assimilative and digestive process, it follows that man is able to come into contact, contain, know, all the individualities of the macrocosm, that is, that man is (or can be) complete mirror of the universe, confirming the analogy, dear to the East and the "esoteric" West, between macrocosm microcosm. Connected to the manipura chakra, the yogis quote the sight. It can be seen that the embryological formation of the optic papillae (extroflexions of the ectodermal cerebral nervous tissue), and subsequently of the eye, occurs only in the presence of a contact between the cupula of the yolk sac (which is the primordial digestive apparatus, endodermal) and the area of optical papillae. It is unusual that the contact is right between the outer leaflet, the ectoderm, and the innermost one, the endoderm. The eye immediately transmits information (ie elements received from the outside) to the brain, whose function of assimilating, containing, transforming, processing information can be considered analogous, albeit on a more "subtle" level, to that of the intestine. Chinese medicine has always emphasized the relationship between the liver (therefore digestive function) and the eye, as belonging to a common "system".

Even for western medicine, the relationship between liver disease and the eye is evident (the yellow eye of the jaundice, the reddened eye of the cirrhotic). Finally, the view is undoubtedly the meaning that allows one to "ingest" the greatest number of details of the external world at the same time (at least for the man in whom the other senses have faded) to allow the brain to "assimilate" them. This chakra is a sort of "control unit" that controls the metabolic functions (especially pancreas and liver) of food and energy; it is therefore linked not only to the transformation of food, but also to the absorption of prana (the mouth that breathes) and to the "metabolization" of all external stimuli and emotions (anxiety, fear, anguish, depression) which are then transmitted to the brain.

Rudra

At the Hindu religion, Rudra ("the screaming one") is one of the oldest pre-Vedic deities.

It appears for the first time in the Rig Veda, in which it is described as the Deva of the storm, of hunting, of death, of nature and of the wind.

Rudra is the primordial form of Śiva, the divine aspect in charge of destruction, and is also a name of Siva in Śiva sahasranama (the repetition of the 1,000 names of Siva).

Rudra, the storm deva, is usually portrayed as a fierce and destructive deity whose terrible darts cause death and disease to humans and beasts. Rudra is currently one of the names of Shiva; the same happens for another epithet, Kapardin (with the spiral braided hair like that of a shell). Rudra is provided with arrows that cause illness in anyone he strikes, whether it be a celestial being, a man or an animal. With Diti he generated the Maruts. The famous hymn Shri Rudram is a Vedic mantra recited today. According to the commentaries to the Vishnu Sahasranama of Adi Sankara, Rudra means "the one who at the time of cosmic dissolution causes all living beings to cry".

Alternatively, Rudra would mean "the one who gives the word". Rudra also means "the one who takes pain away".

How to activate the 3rd chakra

- Open yourself to the energy of the Sun, sunbathe (even if dosed) and recharge yourself with the heat of the sun.
- Add the yellow color to your life, using clothes of that color or surround yourself with yellow upholstery at home.
- Mingle on the fire element: sit down by the fireplace or around the campfire, or light a candle at home.
- The open "O" vowel stimulates the chakra: while seated, inhale and vibrate the open "O" while exhaling, performing the exercise for at least 5 minutes.
- Enjoy sufficient amounts of heat, keep warm especially in winter, have a sauna and practice sports.
- The music that involves the senses strengthens the third chakra so choose Chopin, Schubert and Brahms pieces or listen to soul or modern music according to your preferences.
- Learn to express your emotions take theater lessons or follow a seminar on body language.

Color of the third chakra

For chromotherapy, but not only, yellow is a vital color that underlines the search for the new. This power that distinguishes yellow in chromotherapy is used in different circumstances of psychophysical discomfort, apathy and depression. Yellow seems to be even more effective in situations of eating disorder, in cases of inappetence and chronic anorexia, as the specific chromatic vibrations are able to stimulate the metabolism and the sense of hunger. The use of yellow stimulates the rationality and the left side of the brain, also improving the gastric functions and toning the lymphatic system. Helps to eliminate toxins through the liver and intestines. In ancient Egypt this color was associated with the God of the Sun, which represented strength and vitality. In China, however, it was a color associated with the spirituality and sacredness of the Buddha.

- Yellow brings relaxation where there is tension in the musculature due to nervousness, tension, fear, anxiety.
- Indicated for people who feel lack of involvement have desire for control and deep insecurity. It stimulates mental activity and brings trust and security, giving joy.
- Being a stimulating color, it should be avoided instead in cases of hysteria and in acute inflammatory states (colitis, gastritis).

- Effects on the psyche: constituent of the nervous system is a strong stimulator of joy, sense of well-being, extroversion and conscious lucidity.

It is a "hot" type energy.
Yellow is lighter than red and therefore more suggestive than stimulating so that its impulse acts in flashes. Yellow is the color of emotional detachment and as such, it also helps us to take work issues more lightly, lightening the stress load.

- Who favors the color Yellow is an extrovert person who welcomes the news with joy and is usually endowed with a fervent imagination. Those who prefer the color Yellow show a vitality in alternating phases with more or less high peaks. Very prolific in terms of ideas that applies to the real world is also subject to rapid changes in the face. He has many expectations about his future and loves renewing himself and making new experiences. He often tends to seek the approval of the people around him and does his best to be admired. Also suffers loneliness.
- Those who shy away from the Yellow color often feel disappointed in their expectations and little esteemed by the people who are part of his circle of acquaintances. It often falls into the trap of the lack of confidence in its means even if this gap can be filled even just by re-accumulating lost energy.

Yellow is the color of the 3rd chakra.

The third chakra is called the solar plexus chakra, or the navel chakra. In Sanskrit language it is called Manipura, which means city of jewels. It has as its symbol a yellow lotus flower with ten petals, on which are the letters Dam, Dham, Nam, Tam, Tham, Dam, Dham, Nam, Pam, Pham.

At the center of the flower are the red triangle of Fire (Tejas), the syllable/root "Ram" and a ram, traditional messenger of Agni, the Hindu Lord of Fire. It is placed in the solar plexus/dome of the diaphragm. From the psycho-energetic point of view, its most important function is related to the personal affirmation and the exercise of individual power with respect to the social and the environment in general; it indicates the realization of the person, how much the person sees his desire for life achievable, how much a person wants and wants to fight for himself, how much a person loves himself.

It develops from 4/6 years until the end of childhood, around 10/12 years, allowing the boy/girl to gain independence and realize emotional separation from parents.

The main pathologies expressed by the third Chakra concern all metabolic diseases, such as diabetes, hyperlipidaemia, liver failure, cirrhosis, gastric and duodenal ulcers, glucose levels, and all pathologies concerning the processes of nutrition, digestion and assimilation. . From the psycho-energetic point of view it is at the level of this Chakra that the emotional forces directed towards the external environment are generated: the feelings of friendship, resentment, sympathy, antipathy.

The third chakra, in particular, is the expression of the awareness that each has of himself: that ability to feel pleasure in knowing how satisfied, but also the humility that distinguishes the one who knows he can always improve, because growth resides in change. It is the Chakra of individual will, charisma and efficiency.

It is the foundation of the social personality.

Excessive functioning causes incapacity to remain calm, outbursts of anger, hyperactivity, stomach disorders of nervous origin; the lacking functioning, on the other hand, causes little energy, shyness, continuous need to resort to exciters or stimulants.

The disharmonic functioning of this Chakra generates the unbridled desire of power, of manipulation, in order to overturn reality always and in its favor; tendentially we can notice a hyperactive attitude, which is put in place to hide the sense of inadequacy and emptiness that is caused by the impotence to manage the situations of absolute power that one would expect to exercise. The inner serenity will be strongly compromised and, obviously, the satisfaction of material wellbeing will be the main one, even at the expense of any pleasant feeling, even coming to consider them undesirable and annoying.

The subject who suffers from a decompensation of the third Chakra is led to lose control of his emotions and develop a strongly aggressive attitude, necessary not to allow others to strip their inner weakness, this would unmask the power games of to whom this subject lives, creating a situation of energetic paralysis that would express itself as desperate and desperate impotence.

An example of this defeated subject can be given by the image of those generally middle-aged people, but increasingly young people, who spend their time in annihilating and destructive activities, such as drinking, using drugs more or less less recognized as such, and generally have a strongly aggressive and overbearing attitude in the family.

In fact, these are followed by a highly depressive situation. In this case the subject will have as main objective the being accepted and welcomed by others, and to achieve this purpose he will deny himself to conform to the way of thinking of the people he wishes to please, suffocating and completely denying his own desires and emotions; nevertheless, on the contrary, precisely because of this frustrating attitude, the arrogance and harassment of members of one's family will increase. Powerful and solar chakra, reveals to everyone their right to exist and their place in the Universe, promoting self-acceptance.

Through its totally harmonic expression, the human being is in the world with the fullness of his physical and mental attributes and allows him to act on the material plane in a loose and harmonious way, promoting the enjoyment of everything. If the third chakra is not perfectly harmonious it can nourish one's sense of inferiority; they can diminish their real mental abilities, such as logic and rationality, and increase, therefore, confusion and a sense of insecurity. It may happen that it feeds its own desire for power, possession and, consequently, even overpowering others to obtain and excel. Will and power represent for everyone, in the current society (especially Western), one of the keys to success, but can represent, when understood in an egoic sense of possession and hoarding, the impossibility of conscious access to the other chakras and, therefore, to a real fullness of one's own Being.

It would be linked to the stomach, intestine, liver, gallbladder, spleen, pancreas. It would stop because of great scares (with stomach contraction) or because of reaction to situations or people that are not accepted and this block would cause incapacity to remain calm, outbursts of anger, hyperactivity, disorders of nervous origin. The element of this chakra is fire.

- The organ of sense related to the manipura are the eyes, seat of the sight, while the action organ is the anus, that is the excretory apparatus (however connected also with muladhara) that directs downwards the produced slags from the process of transformation and assimilation that fire performs.

The main characteristic of this chakra is the heat whereby the concentration operated on it encourages heating and combustion. The choice of the yellow is therefore a search for the new, the change, the liberation from the schemes. Synonymous with liveliness, extroversion, lightness, growth and change. He who wears yellow feels good with himself; it is, in fact, the color associated with the sense of identity, with the ego, with extroversion.

Always denotes a strong personality, dominant, intellectual, courageous, responsible, insecure, coordinated, sociable and friendly. It is contraindicated in all situations of excessive nervousness and irritability, acute palpitation and dysentery. Yellow foods such as lemons, grapefruits, oranges, peppers, melons, pineapples, yellow plums, bananas, vegetable oils are the richest in vitamin C which strengthens the immune system and has a purifying effect on the whole organism. They also contain two antioxidants, zeaxanthin and lutein, which strengthen eyesight. And then, plenty of carotene, essential for protecting cells from aging. Yellow is cheerful, raises morale and conveys joy in every environment.

It is the lightest color of the color scale and has a reviving effect on every room, even in the purest and most intense shades. The yellow fills the sunny house regardless of the tones you have chosen: warm as saffron, sunflower, ocher or cold like lemon yellow, primrose or butter. Yellow is the ideal color if you want a room full of light and sunrays: even cool colors such as greens and blues become warmer, and the most interesting neutral colors. It is no coincidence that lemon yellow and ocher prevail in Provence.

Some shades of yellow give a warm feeling and shine like gold. But there are also some colder tones like primrose yellow.

- A garish lemon yellow, especially when matched with a bright green and a light turquoise, communicates energy. Rooms with little light acquire heat and freshness.

The yellow brings warm accents in rather cold environments and enhances details, but can also be used on larger surfaces for its light and bright tones suitable for rooms of all sizes and all light conditions. Yellow increases the attractiveness of sunny rooms and gives warmth and light to the colder ones exposed to the north; this is why yellow is often used, when natural light is scarce. Blue and yellow are a very cheerful combination, evoking joyful visions of sea and sand, sunflowers and summer sky. An intense egg yellow is a strong color and requires strong combinations. It is beautiful with navy blue and a fresh green leaf. Blue-gray, mint green and sugar paper are best combined with primrose yellow and butter-colored. Yellow should be used in meeting and conference rooms and in classrooms to promote better communication. It is also suitable in the dining room or in the living room due to its natural vitality, capable of creating a comfortable and welcoming atmosphere.

Indications:
- Bronchitis

- Spleen: exerts an inhibitory function on the spleen, acts as a purgative, regularizes the flow of bile, fights the parasites.
- Aesthetics: it is mainly used in the case of oily, asphyxial, acneic skin and in lymphatic stasis. Its action is restructuring, bio revitalizing and above all antioxidant. It is active often combined with other colors in impure skin with acne tendency, in the asphyxiated epidermis, stressed and lacking in tone. With yellow the functioning of the cells improves and the skin gains in elasticity, freshness and beauty.
- Nervous exhaustion
- Skin poisoning: Yellow irradiation facilitates the disappearance of scars, even from acne.
- Low concentration: Increases efficiency, amplifies communication and expressive skills, encourages concentration and clarity of reasoning, stimulates memory and capacity for reflection. Writing on light yellow sheets helps to clarify the ideas if they are confusing.
- Sedentariness: A twenty-minute irradiation with yellow and the use of solarized water of the same color, serves to maintain the line in sedentary subjects and for those who tend to gain weight.
- Rheumatism.
- Sinusitis.
- Constipation.

Essential oils associated with the third chakra

Sweet orange, Geranium, Juniper, Mint, Grapefruit, Ginger, Bergamot, Lemon, Rosemary activate the third chakra.

Mix each single essential oil with a carrier oil, for example jojoba or almond oil, in a ratio of 2 drops per tablespoon of carrier oil, then 2 drops per 10 ml of carrier. Since this is a "vibrational treatment" a very diluted mixture will have a deeper and more marked action. Massage the chakra on which you want to work with the mixture containing the selected essential oil. Use a few drops and apply them slowly with your fingertips and in a circular motion in a clockwise direction. As you massage the Chakra, focus on the result you want to achieve, displaying the harmonic energy of the oil as it opens and rebalances the chakra. After treatment, stay relaxed and relaxed for a while, allowing the Chakra to rebalance. Breathe deeply and slowly, trying to free and clear your mind as much as possible.

As an alternative to massage, add a few drops of the essential oil chosen for the treatment to the essence diffuser. Focus and focus on your therapeutic intention, visualize the aromatherapy energy of the essential oil, open and rebalance the chakra. Relax for at least half an hour.

Sweet orange

The sweet orange essential oil is popular in aromatherapy for its anxiolytic and calmed properties. In aromatherapy it is used against anxiety and stress. Perfect for use as an air freshener in a student's study room. It is used as a natural remedy for other emotional disorders such as depression and nervousness. The essential oil of orange stimulates the production of bile and accelerates the intestinal peristalsis: its action is therefore effective in counteracting constipation. It has a slightly hypnotic effect, acts as a sedative: it is therefore useful for treating nervous disorders, insomnia. It also fights infections, has diuretic and febrifugal action, is a muscular and nervous tonic, stimulates and strengthens natural defenses.

Moreover the essential oil of orange also acts effectively on the skin; fights wrinkles and facilitates cell turnover; it tightens the tissues and contrasts eczema and dermatosis.

- 300 kg of skins are required to obtain 1 liter of essential oil, with a warm and sweet scent, of a color ranging from orange-yellow to dark-red.

His homeland is China and seems to have been imported into Europe just in the fourteenth century by Portuguese sailors. But some ancient Romans already speak of it in the first century; It was cultivated in Sicily and called it melarancia, which could mean that the fruit had reached Europe by land. The ancient technique of extracting the essential oil of sweet orange was called nuance. The shaders were very skilled craftsmen who cut the fruit into two parts by rubbing the outer portion of the peel onto a sponge. In doing so they broke the vesicles that are found on the peel of the fruit, collecting the essential oil that came out, the water contained in the peel and little juice that dripped. Their ability was to exert the right pressure, so as not to pour too much juice and proceed quickly with the work. Then the sponges were squeezed into a container for collection.

The liquid, left to rest, divided and the upper part was constituted by the essential oil, lighter than water and insoluble in it. Today the work of the nuances is carried out by machines called shading machines and the separation of the two liquids is done by centrifugation.

This method makes it possible to obtain a prized oil more easily, without the use of chemical solvents.

- Part used: the skin also called peel.
- Extraction method: cold pressing of fresh fruits.
- Top note: sweet, fresh, fruity bouquet.

Relaxing bath: It is considered a mild sedative and used to fight insomnia in a natural way. Before going to bed, indulge in a long relaxing bath in a hot tub with 15 drops of sweet orange essence to be emulsified with Dead Sea salts (or common cooking salt) and shaking well before diving.

Shower: 3-4 drops on a wet terry glove gently massage the whole body.

Environmental diffusion: 1 drop of sweet orange essential oil for every square meter of the environment in which it spreads, through the burner of essential oils or in the water of the radiator humidifiers.

Contraindications: For external use only. Its prolonged use on the skin species of the face may be poorly indicated, should not be used before exposure to sunlight for tanning, it would make the skin sensitive and prone to cracking or even severe burns.

Geranium

In aromatherapy the essential oil of geranium is used in cases of acne, anxiety, depression, stress, insomnia and sore throat. The essential oil of geranium has antibacterial, antidepressive, anti-inflammatory, antiseptic, astringent, diuretic, repellent and tonic properties. This makes it suitable for use for numerous health and wellness issues. It is also used to promote emotional stability, to relieve pain thanks to its pain-relieving properties, to stimulate the healing of burns and wounds thanks to its healing properties, to improve mood and reduce inflammation. It is useful to perform massages at the level of the legs to reactivate the circulation.

- Originally from South Africa, geranium was introduced into Europe in the seventeenth century by British and Dutch settlers, who, on their return from the Indies, stopped with their ships at Cape of Good Hope to obtain supplies.

In our continent it began to be cultivated, especially in the Mediterranean belt, which has a climate similar to that of its origin. The geranium is composed of hundreds of different species, each characterized by its own colors, intensity of scent, petals and degree of resistance to temperatures. In the past it was widely used to combat bleeding due to its strong astringent and healing action; today it is very widespread, especially as an ornamental plant and its essential oil is used by the cosmetics industry and by the food and liquor industry.

The oil that is extracted from the geranium, just distilled, looks like a green liquid with a sweet and very delicate smell, which is then processed and mixed according to need or left in its pure state.

- Part used: leaves and flowers.
- Extraction method: steam distillation
- Heart note: fresh, sweet, floral scent.

Rebalancing: it is used in aromatherapy to increase imagination and intuition so as to be able to find solutions in tangled or difficult situations. It stimulates the desire and the desire to express oneself and to bring out what is felt in the deep, helps to become aware and to balance the give-have. Very suitable for people who do not know what they want stimulates their motivation. Attract to us all that is positive. It helps to promote sleep and relaxation. You can apply a few drops on a handkerchief to be placed on the bedside table or to be kept close to the pillow, or have a massage in the neck and shoulders before going to sleep.

Toning: indicated in massages to reactivate blood circulation, to combat cellulite, and in treatment, prevention or normalization of disorders that originate from a malfunction of the circulatory system, such as varicose veins, capillary and couperose fragility. The essential oil of geranium is considered useful for preventing and relieving wrinkles. That's why it is used as an ingredient in anti-aging creams. You can add a single drop of geranium essential oil to the moisturizer that is usually used for the face. As after sun, dilute 5 drops of Geranium essential oil, 5 of Chamomile and 1 of Peppermint in a spoon of Jojoba Oil and add to the bath and / or rub before going to sleep.

Contraindications: The essential oil of geranium is considered safe, so there are no special precautions to be followed. It is important to remember that the improper use of essential oils can be harmful, so always rely on the advice of an herbalist.

Bergamot

Some derive its name from the Turkish beg armudi = "pear of God", due to its similarity to the shape of the bergamotta pear; others from the city of Bergamo where its oil was first sold. The exact genesis of this citrus is not known, the yellow color would indicate a derivation by genetic mutation starting from pre-existent citrus species such as lemon, bitter orange or lime. Some legends see it originally from the Canary Islands, from which it was imported by Christopher Columbus, other sources tend to China, Greece, or the city of Berga in Spain.

One of these legends tells the story of the Moor of Spain, who sold a branch, for eighteen scudi, to the gentlemen Valentino di Reggio Calabria, who grafted it on a bitter orange, in one of their estates in the district "Santa Caterina". In this province the bergamot has one of its best habitats: in no other part of the world there is a place where this citrus fruit with the same yield and quality of essence.

Bergamot is a citrus fruit that probably derives from a cross between bitter orange and sour lime, although many consider it a real species called Citrus bergamia Risso (of Chinese origin). Its presence in Calabria is presumable between the fourteenth and the sixteenth century. In 1750 the first "bergamotteto" would have been planted around it.

- 90% of the total production of bergamot comes from Calabria, in Italy. The essential oils of bergamot, by virtue of their extraordinary fragrance, are used in the industrial production of perfumes, sweets and liqueurs. It is an essence that, thanks to its freshness, represents the basic element for the production of numerous colognes and cosmetics.

In fact, even if it is cultivated in the Ivory Coast, Argentina, Brazil, the quality of the obtained essence is not comparable with that of the Calabrian bergamot, in Italy.

- Its cultivation has developed above all for the production of perfumes and more generally in the cosmetic industry. In the city of Cologne, Paolo Feminis started producing the Aqua admirabilis, a scent based on bergamot. The real development in the production of perfume, however, is due to one of his nephew, Gian Maria Farina, Italian emigrant, who in 1704 started the production of the Water of Cologne in that city.

Whatever its history or the etymology of its name, the essential oil of bergamot, has long been used in folk medicine, for the treatment of fever, including malaria, and for intestinal parasites.

- Part used - peel of almost ripe fruit.
- Extraction method - cold pressing.

- Top note: soft, fresh, fruity and slightly balsamic scent.

Antidepressant: in aromatherapy it is used to combat stress and to reduce agitation, confusion, depression and fear, showing optimism and serenity. If inhaled, it induces a joyful and dynamic mood, eliminating psychological blocks. It makes it possible to give and receive love, to radiate happiness around oneself and to care for others. Add 8 drops to 30-40 ml of jojoba oil or sweet almond and gently massage, with circular movements, the temples or, alternatively, two drops on the handkerchief, to be inhaled when needed.

Calming: acts on the nervous system by contrasting anxiety, it is an effective remedy in case of insomnia, because it relaxes, reconciling sleep.

Contraindications: the essential oil of bergamot is very valuable and therefore easily prone to counterfeits; it is cut with synthetic or poor quality essences. It is important that the choice falls on quality products that repay in terms of benefits, oil must be pure.
The essential oil of bergamot must never be used pure because it is very concentrated and can be too aggressive due to the presence of terpenes.
Its effectiveness is enhanced if diluted in a carrier substance, at a concentration never higher than 1% (about 3 or 4 drops per 100 ml).

The essential oil of bergamot is phototoxic, so if applied to the skin avoid sun exposure.

Furocumarins, such as bergaptene, cause sensitization and pigmentation on the skin, following exposure to direct sunlight. A precaution is therefore necessary if the oil is applied to the skin. Apart from this the essential oil of bergamot is non-toxic and non-irritating. Do not use during pregnancy, lactation and in young children. The essential oil of bergamot must be protected from sunlight, because bergaptene, one of its components, becomes toxic if exposed to sunlight.

Juniper

Known for its many properties, it is useful for the circulatory system and disorders such as back pain or muscle pain. One of the main properties of this plant is to be a powerful detoxifier. Its oil is excellent for promoting drainage and elimination of cell catabolites (toxins). Its activity is favorably expressed at the level of lymphatic circulation, promoting the elimination of waste through diuresis.

Its action against pain and relieving rheumatism and arthritis is now well known, as is also recognized its effectiveness on tendinitis, fascitis and muscle contractures, especially in the field of physiotherapy and sports. Together with the devil's claw and essential oil of eucalyptus, juniper can be applied, with a decontracting sports massage, on the contracted muscles in order to relax dissolve tension and contractures and bring benefits to tense and aching muscles. From the distillation of the Juniper, liquors such as gin, grappa and super-alcohol are obtained.

Its berries are widely used in cooking to season game, in order to cover the smell of game and make them even more digestible. Like all strongly aromatic plants, juniper and its derivatives have an aperitif and stimulating action of the epigastric function. Known since ancient times especially for its purifying and antiseptic properties, its branches were burned to disinfect ships from areas where epidemics had occurred; something that is still done today in the breeding of silkworms, to purify the shelters of insects. From the distillation of its berries, a strong liqueur called "gin" is obtained. The juniper was and still is, a plant appreciated by mountaineers to flavor grappa and roasts. The hunters know very well that the thrushes are fond of juniper galbula and that their meat takes on for this reason a particularly delicious flavor.

- Part used: green berries and young branches.
- Extraction method: steam distillation. It is carried out in the coldest periods of the year to reduce the loss of active ingredients by evaporation which is greater in the hot months.
- Base note: fresh, sweet, balsamic scent.

Anti-inflammatory: it is used with benefit against headaches, rheumatic pains, arthrosis, arthritis, gout and other inflammations of the osteoarticular system: rubbing on the painful part a mixture of essential oil and vegetable oil, the body's production of cortisone is stimulated, with a marked analgesic effect.

Relaxation: excellent decontracting for the muscular system and tendon loosens the muscles and is especially indicated for athletes after physical activity or in case of tension, pain and back pain and stress.

46

Relaxing bath: place 12 drops of juniper essential oil in the tub water. Stay immersed in the tub, in the dark, for at least twenty minutes.

This bath is more effective if done in the evening, before going to bed against rheumatism and muscle pain.

Contraindications: For external use only. The essential oil of juniper should never be applied directly to the skin, because it can irritate. It is forbidden to use Juniper during pregnancy as it performs a stimulating action on the smooth muscles, with consequent contraction of the uterine walls; instead it is recommended to use it in the postpartum period to favor the closure of the cervix.

It is never advisable for internal use of this essential oil without strict medical supervision, however in no case in the presence of kidney disease.

Mint

Mint oil has many properties and its use proves beneficial, to combat different problems, such as gastrointestinal problems, rheumatic pains, dermatological disorders. It is also effective for counteracting all symptoms of flu and cold and helps with anxiety and insomnia. Among the uses there is also that for cosmetics, thanks to the fact that the essential oil of peppermint has excellent refreshing properties.

- The name "mint" comes from the Greek Mintha, a nymph daughter of Cocito, one of the five rivers of the Underworld, loved by Pluto and transformed into a plant by the goddess Persephone, his bride.

According to mythology, the goddess discovered the betrayal of her husband and, seized by an impetus of jealousy, wanted to take revenge by turning it into a seemingly insignificant and inconspicuous seedling, relegating it to grow near the banks of the paternal river, near the waters. However, in order not to disdain altogether Pluto allowed the seedling to still have something pleasant in every part of his body: the fresh aroma of his perfume. Already Pliny enumerated all his properties, exalting the fragrance, "able to excite the soul and stimulate the appetite".

The mint-based preparations, according to the Roman historian, healed the tonsillar angina, the blood spitting of tuberculosis, the sob, the vomit, and helped to eliminate the parasites. In the 18th century Nicolò Lemery, in his Treatise on Simple Drugs, presented his interpretation of the allegedly exciting and tonic virtues of the plant: "Mentha is dedicated to the mind because this plant fortifying the brain, awakens thoughts or memory".

- Part used: leaves and top.
- Extraction method: steam distillation.
- Top note: fresh, strong, sweet-bitter, pungent scent.

Antistress: if inhaled, has a refreshing and regenerating effect on the psyche. It is effectively used to promote concentration during the study for exams, or to improve office performance. The essential oil of mint also has a toning action, useful in case of psycho-physical fatigue and neurovegetative problems, due to states of stress, such as anxiety, insomnia, depression.

Environmental diffusion: 1 drop of essential oil of mint, for every square meter of the environment in which it spreads, through a burner of essential oils or in the water of the radiator humidifiers, for a regenerating and purifying effect in smoking rooms and in who studies.

Antiemetic: the soothing properties of this essence help to reduce the discomfort of nausea and vomiting, for this reason it is advisable to have the essential oil of mint always at hand during travel, to counteract the car sickness.

Contraindications: Do not apply pure essential oil of mint to the skin, but always mix it with a base oil (Jojoba oil, sweet almond oil). It is not suitable for children under the age of 12.

It is advisable that those who follow a homeopathic treatment avoid the use of the essential oil of peppermint, because interactions may occur. Pay attention to the eyes, as it is highly irritating to the mucous membranes. Do not exceed the recommended dose.

Grapefruit

Known for its many properties, it has a balancing, toning effect on the muscles and slimming on the accumulation of fats. Grapefruit essential oil is excellent for the composition of ointments to be used for anti-cellulite massages. Grapefruit is an ancient hybrid, probably between sweet orange and pomelo, but has for centuries been an autonomous species that propagates by cuttings and grafting.

The industry derives essential oils from the peel; to get 1 kg of grapefruit essence you need 200 kg of peel, about 2,000 grapefruits.

Grapefruit is the only citrus that is supposed not to come from Southeast Asia, but from Central America. It is said to have been discovered in 1750, probably in Barbadoso in the Bahamas. There are no certain data about it, but there is the hypothesis that grapefruit also came to Europe together with its progenitor, sweet orange, from the Far East through Asia to the Silk Road, which would place the its origin in the homeland of all the other citrus fruits. The fruit only became popular in the nineteenth century.

- Part used: fruit rind.
- Extraction method: mechanical pressing.
- Top note: citrus scent, delicately fresh, bitter.

Rebalancing: if inhaled, stimulates and revitalizes the body, infusing a new energetic charge. Promotes the proper function of the endocrine glands, especially the hypothalamus, in the production of regulatory hormones of the primary functions of the organism, such as the sleep/wake cycle, hunger/satiety, and those that intervene on the stability of mood. For this reason it is indicated in the treatment of nervous hunger, in seasonal changes, to facilitate the adaptation of the organism to climate changes, to overcome jet lag, during periods of nervous exhaustion, anxiety or severe stress due to unbalanced life rhythms.

This regulatory action of the hormonal system also has the effect of increasing the immune system. It has the characteristic of acting on the nervous center that regulates the appetite or its lack, in cases of anorexia and bulimia, take 1 drop at the 3 meals on bread or honey. To purify the blood and fortify the immune system during the spring or autumn period, drink 1 cup of nettle tea with 1 drop of grapefruit essence and 1 teaspoon of honey, every day, for a period of 4 weeks.

Relaxing bath: pour 10-20 drops into the water of the tub, emulsify by shaking the water strongly, then immerse yourself for 10 minutes to stimulate the lymphatic circulation, tone and relax the muscles, after intense sports, or to relax in case of nervousness and stress.

Environmental diffusion: 1 drop of essential oil of grapefruit, for every square meter of the environment in which it spreads, through the burner of essential oils or in the water of the radiator humidifiers in case of depression or nervous breakdown and to cool the air.

Massage oil: mix 20 drops of grapefruit essential oil in 100 ml. sweet almond oil and gently massage the affected areas until completely absorbed, in the presence of cellulite, water retention or localized adiposity and to firm the skin and underlying tissues. To prepare an ointment for anti-cellulite massages, add 3 drops of essential oil of grapefruit, 2 drops of essential oil of cypress, 2 drops of essential oil of rosemary, 2 drops of essential oil of sweet orange, a tablespoon of almond oil .

- Rosemary essential oil stimulates blood circulation by performing a perfect action to counteract water retention.
- The essential oil of cypress includes astringent and tonic properties.
- Grapefruit essential oil promotes the drainage of toxic substances.

Contraindications: Like all essential oils, grapefruit is a very concentrated substance that should not be used pure, but always diluted in a solvent or carrier oil. Avoid contact with eyes and mucous membranes. Do not exceed the recommended daily dose. Keep out of reach of children under the age of 3. During treatment with this essence, avoid prolonged exposure to the sun, as a photosensitizer. Contraindicated in pregnancy and lactation.

Ginger

The spicy and tasty ginger gives us the essential oil of ginger: invigorating and aphrodisiac, with beneficial actions on the whole organism. Known for its many properties, it is useful in cases of nausea, anxiety, headaches and colds. The essential oil of ginger is also seen as an excellent natural remedy against cellulite. Ginger has been used in the East for thousands of years, both for flavoring and flavoring food, and as a medicinal remedy for various ailments.

- In Thailand, ginger root compresses and compresses are applied, crushed and mixed with other herbs, for the painful articular and muscular states very frequent in the environments of Muay Thai, the art of Thai boxing.

Ginger is also used for its dynamizing and energizing power, in all conditions of weakness and physical exhaustion. In Traditional Chinese Medicine the root is called gan-jiang and is considered an effective Yang tonic, used to strengthen the male energies, fire and vitality, to treat male impotence and asthenia. In Ayurvedic medicine, it is connected to the Fire element, linked to the functionality of the spleen. Even today in many Asian countries the fresh rhizome is used in the states of fatigue, to relieve toothaches, rheumatic pains, colds, malaria and all those that are called "wet states" such as diarrhea or excess of mucus. In the ancient West, Greeks and Romans imported ginger from the Red Sea area and knew its important medicinal properties, as well as using it as a spice.

In the Middle Ages the legendary Hildegard abbess of Bingen, mystical and herbalist of the 11th century, advised to macerate it in wine and make compresses for eye disorders or to drink a glass of ginger wine sweetened with honey to promote vitality in convalescents and in the elderly.

- Part used: deboned and dried rhizome.
- Extraction method: steam distillation.
- Base note: warm, spicy, pungent scent.

Toning on the whole organism: if inhaled, it rebalances the energies that are not in harmony. It helps to awaken and warm the dormant senses, improves concentration and the ability to discern. At the aromatherapy level, the essence of ginger acts against fatigue, weakness and nervous exhaustion; it gives courage and helps to react by eliminating confusion and despair. It stimulates openness to the outside, generating new interests. At a mental level, it favors concentration and helps to undo psychological knots. It is an essence that gives energy and vitality.

Anti-nausea: useful for preparing for long and tiring journeys, because anxiety decreases; it is used as a moderator in motion sicknesses (passive movement disorders such as air, sea and car sickness), and against the growth hormone nausea present in the first months of gestation. The disturbances of seasickness, car or plane disappear simply by smelling the aroma of 2-3 drops of essential oil of ginger during the journey that we will have poured on a handkerchief.

Massage oil: in 200 ml of sweet almond oil put 40 drops, massage 2-3 times a day the painful area, or the belly in case of slow digestion, in the presence of intestinal gas and diarrhea.

Contraindications: No contraindications.
However, before taking the product for internal use, consult an herbalist; like all essential oils, in fact, it can be irritating to the mucous membranes. The essential oil of ginger is photosensitive and, in case of skin application, it is not recommended sun exposure in the following 12 hours. Furthermore, since it promotes bile release, essential ginger oil is not recommended for those suffering from gallstones. It is advised not to use it to reduce nausea during pregnancy and pure on the skin.

Lemon

Lemon essential oil has an antiseptic, antibiotic, purifying, balancing, hemostatic and healing action on small wounds, ulcers, cold sores, gingival inflammation. In particular, the antibiotic action of limonene in combination with the antioxidant vitamin C gives the lemon the ability to increase the immune system and to fight problems such as sore throat, cough, and flu symptoms.

The essential oil of lemon, because of its high intake of vitamin C and B vitamins, is a useful ally to combat the signs of aging: it reduces wrinkles, stimulates cell regeneration of the skin, accelerates the disappearance of Acne and strengthens the nails. It must be emphasized that vitamin PP, in particular, activates venous and lymphatic circulation, with beneficial effects on cellulite, on circulatory problems in the legs, on capillary fragility, on strengthening vessels, on blood thinning.

The essential oil of lemon is also an adjuvant in the treatment of hypertension, arthritis, rheumatism. Thanks to the citrates contained in it, the lemon essential oil also encourages digestion, stimulates the functioning of the liver and pancreas, eliminates acidity and burns.

- The ancient Greeks called the lemon "apple of Media" because they came from Media, a country near Persia. At that time it was only used to perfume clothes and the numerous therapeutic properties were not known.

When we talk about essential oils obtained from citrus fruits we can use the term "essences"; in fact, with the terms "lemon essence" and "lemon essential oil", the same product extracted from the fruit is indicated. The lemon essential oil is obtained only from the lemon peel, which is richer in active substances, and preferably from non-fully ripe fruit. It looks like a yellowish liquid, with a slightly bitter but very fragrant taste. To produce a few milliliters of essential oil you need several kilos of lemons.

- Part used: peel.
- Extraction method: cold pressing.
- Top note: citrus, sweet, fruity bouquet.

Calming: on the psyche and on the nervous system the essential oil of lemon, if inhaled, helps in case of anxiety disorders, nervousness that causes headaches or insomnia and improves memory. It prevents blockages of the sympathetic nervous system, stimulates parasympathetic functions. It supports, instills courage and determination. When one is forced to suffer oppression, persecution and harassment of various kinds, helps to free oneself from conditioning.

Massage oil: in 250 ml of sweet almond oil, put 15 drops of lemon essential oil. Massage the legs from the ankles to the pelvis in case of capillary fragility cellulitis or varicose veins.

Contraindications: The essential oil of lemon is non-toxic, but it can irritate the skin or give sensitization reactions in particular predisposed subjects. It is however toxic photo, so it should not be used on the skin if it is subsequently exposed directly to the sun or tanning lamps. It is not recommended in case of hypotension: prolonged and excessive use of the essential lemon oil can cause pressure drop and collapse.

Any use you want to make lemon essential oil, it is important that it is always pure, without synthetic substances. In case of internal use, the daily dose to be used should not exceed a few drops, mixed with teas, water, honey.

Rosemary

Rosemary is popular for its stimulating and purifying properties, its essential oil has always been used for its cardiotonic and anti-cellulite properties. Rosemary essential oil has interesting anti-dandruff properties, is perfect for the natural treatment of oily hair, skin care, solar eczema and to relieve muscle pain.

- Rosemary essential oil is widely used in aromatherapy, so much so as to be included among the essential oils that can never be lacking in the home.

On a physical level, rosemary has strong purifying powers, helps eliminate toxins and excess water. For skin care can be used to dab in the case of acne and eczema, to perfume face creams and is recommended especially in the case of oily skin.

The massage with rosemary essential oil relieves arthritic and muscular pains, dissolves uric acid and crystals that harden the epidermal tissues. Its stimulating action also acts on the urinary tract: it favors diuresis and is therefore indicated in case of renal failure. Rosemary has a beneficial action on the gland by stimulating the function of the liver and the excretion of bile. Thanks to these properties it is used effectively in diseases of the liver and of the gallbladder in general. The Egyptians knew the bactericidal and antiseptic effects of this essence and used it in the tombs.

Even in Greece its twigs were burned in the temples instead of the precious Arab incense.

The Ancient Romans used to cultivate rosemary on the tombs, as a symbol of immortality. In the Middle Ages, an edict of Charlemagne of 812 forced the peasants to cultivate in the gardens a rosemary plant, whose scent was believed to contain the soul of the earth; while in popular tradition it was used against plague and infectious diseases.

- Part used: leaves, flowering tops, twigs.
- Extraction method: steam distillation.
- Base note, woody, balsamic, camphor fragrance.

Stimulating: on the nervous system if inhaled, gives energy, promotes concentration and improves memory, especially during periods of intense pressure for intellectual activities. When used in the morning it has a general toning action; dissolves and stimulates our emotional components, infuses courage, reinforces the will. True enemy of illusions teaches us to look away and to clearly perceive the nuances of life. To strengthen self-confidence and self-esteem, in the morning shower add 3-4 drops of rosemary essential oil to a dose of neutral liquid soap.

Environmental diffusion: 1 drop of rosemary essential oil, for every square meter of the environment in which it spreads, through a burner of essential oils or in the water of the radiator humidifiers to cool and deodorize the air and promote concentration.

Toning bath: dilute 10-15 drops of essence in a tub of water to calm and neutralize tension, fight stress and rheumatism, muscle aches, arthritis, bruises and sciatica.

Contraindications: Rosemary essential oil is not irritating, but should always be used diluted, and should not be used for long periods. Pay attention to the quantities because in high doses in indoor use it can be toxic. Contraindicated in pregnancy, in epileptic subjects and for children. An abuse causes dangerous effects on the organism: gastrointestinal and urinary tract disorders are possible; it can also be convulsive and cause insomnia if used in the evening hours.

Himalayan flowers for the third chakra

The Himalayan Enhancers Flowers directly influence the various levels of energy controlled by the Chakras, removing negative feelings and stimulating positive ones. The Himalayan Flowers Enhancers were identified by Tanmaya in 1990, during a stay of several months in a Himalayan valley.

The term Enhancers means catalysts, because the essences are not only remedies aimed at working on negative emotions and inner states but also encourage processes of energetic rebalancing and spiritual development that are very profound to bring to light qualities buried within the person.

They can be hired alone or diluted together with Bach Flowers or other Flowers.

The first preparations of Tanmaya concerned nine combinations, seven directly related to the plexuses, better known by the Indian name of chakra plus a general catalyst and a flower particularly suitable for children; subsequently their number has multiplied with the discovery of new flowers, suitable for modulating specific emotions.

They are Flowers with a very quick and powerful effect, unlike the Bach Flowers, which are among the slowest and most delicate; this power is sometimes very useful, other times it can represent a risk of excessive action. While Bach Flowers can be considered primarily emotional remedies, ie aimed at rebalancing human emotions, the Himalayan Flowers, thanks to the nature of the soil on which they grow, are essentially addressed to the spiritual dimension of man, stimulating the need for prayer, of meditation and connection with the divine who dwells in him.

- Himalayan flower essences are liquid extracts that contain the energy of the flower to be administered generally by mouth, they can also be used in the bath water, nebulized on the body or in the environment, or combined with the oil for massage.

Strength

It helps to develop individuality, creativity, sincerity, honesty, self-esteem.

Love, identification and ability to manifest oneself. Helps overcome the lack of self-confidence, doubts, the inability to express one's innate creativity. Dissolves the sense of insecurity, the voids of personal power, the lack of directives in life, motivations, hope, eliminates depression, oppression. It helps to get rid of the patterns that compel and condition.

There are moments in life when we feel shy, we are afraid to act, fear of the judgment of others, we do not do what we really want, but only what others expect from us, we can not say no, we are afraid to defend our ideas, we are afraid to disappoint, that others do not want us any more. We are dominated by feelings of guilt. Or we feel melancholy, sad, unable to act, inert, we do not know which direction to take even if we know that what we are following is not the right one. Strength helps to set concrete goals and implement them in real life, to give meaning and direction to one's life, to increase one's personal power.

When in the third chakra there are blocks or weaknesses, there is a psychic collapse and the person risks succumbing to others and life, becomes timid, passive, frightening and insecure.

The need for security and protection determines involutive mechanisms, in which there is a return to childish behavior.

You can be both timid and irritable, aggressive and fearful, melancholy and hyperactive, sad and happy. The great fear of action and exposure leads to take on the behaviors and mental schemes imposed by society, to conform, to do what everyone does, what must be done. Strength develops individuality, creativity, honesty, self-esteem, our expression in the material world. Love, identification and ability to manifest oneself. Helps overcome the lack of directives, motivations, hope in life, eliminates depression and oppression, free from the mental schemes that compel and condition.

It allows you to overcome stress, the inner tension that is exhausting, the melancholy, the fear that blocks, which does not act, which inhibits and takes away concreteness and courage. Strengthens determination, self-esteem, honesty. The dosage of taking the essences, pure or diluted, is two drops under the tongue several times a day

It helps to develop one's personality and individuality, to get out of social and family patterns, develops one's personal power, one's own strength. He teaches not to do things for others, but for himself, not to worry about the judgment of others, not to be afraid to expose himself, to tell his own truth.

Californian flowers for the third chakra

The Californian Flowers extend the Bach Flowers.
Richard Kats and Patricia Kaminski, founders of the FES (Flower Essence Society), together with the work of other researchers have discovered more than 150 flowers since 1979. They work on specific problems more modern and current and that at the time when Bach lived not they were so preponderant or they did not yet talk about them like today: anorexia and bulimia, sexual disorders, diseases derived from environmental pollution.

It is possible to create composite essences by joining Bach and Californian flowers, as well as essences of other floriterapic repertoires of other parts of the world. The Californian floral remedies are prepared in the same, simple way of the flowers of Bach, placing the corolla of wild flowers in a glass bowl full of spring water and letting them infuse in the sun for a few hours. This liquid, rich in vital force, is then filtered, diluted in brandy and used for the preparation of the so-called stock bottles (or concentrates).

The choice of essences, as happens with Bach flowers, is always personalized and in relation to the state of mind and the emotions that one wants to rebalance. Once you have chosen the remedy or remedies indicated for the personal problem, you pour two drops of ciscuno into a small bottle with a 30 ml dropper, filled with natural mineral water and two teaspoons of brandy as a preservative.

- The dosage is 4 drops 4 times a day, for a period of a few weeks or in any case until the symptoms have improved or disappeared.

Being a completely natural cure and free from toxicity, do not have any contraindication, do not cause side effects, can be combined without problems both traditional and homeopathic medicines (of which they are considered complementary) or to other therapeutic flours remedies.

Blackberry

The characteristic common to all the bramble species is to develop even in difficult habitats and to regrow despite drastic and radical pruning. It therefore represents the ability to struggle to live and fully express its potential. People unable to realize their aspirations and desires or to reach their goals. They lack the willpower, the ability and the energy to realize.

They feel stuck and immobilized, they have a lot of imagination and high desires, but they are not able to concretize them. Generally, they are subjects in which thought is dissociated from the will.

They are people who feel frustrated because of the inability to achieve what they would like or suffer from the inconsistency between their thoughts and actions. They have high ideals, great aspirations, but they lack concreteness, and often also of will and decision-making ability, so not being able to live as they wish they suffer a lot. For all states of lethargy and mental confusion. Awakens latent attitudes.

A help for conception in women who have difficulty. In children to develop interest and involvement in homework and duties at school and home. It allows the thought to go into action. In the group: for those who tend to be idealistic or to have an excessively philosophical vision, but it is hard to commit their will to the group's projects.

These people often have a lot of light surrounding their head, which, however, does not radiate and does not circulate properly throughout the body. Blood circulation is often slow, as is all their lower metabolism.

When the light manages to reach the members, the individual feels greater inner power to act concretely in the world and to translate what is spiritual into a real change in society.

Blackberry floral essence gives this radiant and active light to the will of the human soul.

Larkspur

For those who tend to be too centralized, to have too much responsibility or to give themselves too much importance. It helps to live the leadership to be a leader who knows how to command in harmony with others, who does not abuse his power, but transmits charisma and enthusiasm. True spiritual leadership requires charisma or a contagious enthusiasm.

When in the individual Larkspur a positive identification with his own inner ideals arises, his altruism feeds and inspires others.

This type of command is not, therefore, an energetic power that manipulates others or a forced and oppressive execution of one's responsibilities; it is rather an inner joy that gives energy to others. Larkspur helps those who take a leading position to align their feelings with spiritual ideals.

In this way, the individual learns to spread an inspired charismatic energy that motivates and encourages others.

Quince

For those people with difficulty in accepting their female aspects; hard and unable to open up to the capacity to love and receptivity.

For those who live as love antagonistic love and strength. For women who deny their femininity as a way of demonstrating being strong. Hardness and rigidity of character in affective relationships, difficulty in harmoniously integrating the masculine and feminine energies within oneself, inability to express sweetness, tenderness, affective warmth because the volitional and rational aspect of their personality represses these feelings (the mind that represses the heart).

Women "in career" who can not manage the power in a harmonious way, who can not express the feminine qualities because they are too busy at work. Need to find a "feminine way" in the management of power.

It can also be of great help to the separated parents who have custody of their children, with whom they must in a certain sense cover the maternal and paternal roles at the same time or for all parents who must show their children both the sweet and protective aspect that a firm discipline and objectivity.

Restores women's maternal capacity and confidence in women's power. With Quince essence, the individual learns that true power is love and that true love also confers authority.

Sunflower

Sunflower is the representation of the Sun which, with its harmonious and balanced expression of masculine creative energy, illuminates the individual and cares with his warmth. Particularly suitable for all people who have a problem to radiate this power in a balanced way, so they have a sense of the unbalanced ego, that is in excess or in defect: for those who are too arrogant and presumptuous, it is vain narcissistic (the brilliance of the sun shines with too much force and dazzles, you have to bring out the heat), or for those who underestimate or suffer from inferiority complex, is insecure and always feels inadequate (the shine of the ego is obscured, light must be given to the soul). The person absorbs the lunar qualities of receptivity and nourishment from the mother, while from the father he learns the solar qualities of the radiant, expressive ego.

- This essence takes care of the problems or distortions of the relationship of the individual with the male, often associated with a conflictual or defective relationship with the father in childhood and is equally important for both men and women.

Useful in adolescent issues when there is a conflict with the authority and the father figure. Improve the relationships of parents with their sons. When the Sunflower individual learns how to harness this great solar force within his ego, he is truly able to give a precious gift to other human beings and to the Earth, taking care of it and making healing.

Australian flowers for the third chakra

The Australian Bush Flower (Australian Bush Flower Essences) are today 69 plus 19 Essences created by the combination of Australian Flowers and were introduced by Ian White, Australian biologist and psychologist. They are not yet widely known and used in Italy by the general public, but they are very appreciated by the Floristapeuti and we find Australian flowers inserted in many complexes phytopreparati and homeopathic. They are among the most powerful and widely used flowers after the Bach Flowers, they have a very high energy, one of the highest among the flower remedies. The Australian Aborigines have always used the Flowers to deal with discomforts or emotional imbalances, as they did in ancient Egypt, India, Asia and South America.

The dose, for both adults and children, consists of seven drops to be taken twice a day (morning and evening) under the tongue, or in a little water. The essences should be taken for about twenty days or a month, with the exception of particularly powerful essences.

Being a completely natural cure and free from toxicity, do not have any contraindication, do not cause side effects, can be combined without problems both traditional and homeopathic medicines (of which they are considered complementary) or other remedies floriterapici. You can prepare only one remedy (whose action will then be particularly "targeted", deep and fast), or mix different remedies with each other; in this case it is advisable not to exceed 4 or 5 essences and, if possible, try to choose flowers with similar and synergistic properties to treat a specific problem.

Australian flowers are also very effective in skin application and can be added to creams, gels, massage oils, medicated ointments or diluted in the bath water.

- For a topical treatment the recommended amount is about 7 drops of each remedy chosen, to be mixed in half a cup of cream; 15-20 drops of each essence should be poured into the bathtub.

The duration of treatment always depends on the individual response.

Often a positive reaction is obtained in about two weeks and on average two months are sufficient to rebalance numerous psychophysical problems. Some particularly "powerful" flowers (such as, for example, Waratah) usually exert a very rapid action, even in a few days. Many times, after having resolved an uneasiness or an inner conflict, other emotional imbalances can emerge, which will be treated with the corresponding flowers.

Peach Flower Tea Tree

It is the remedy for those who lack the will to continue something for which initially they had great enthusiasm and that now has left them without interest. Those who are subject to mood swings, moody ups and hypochondria.

The flower helps to find a renewed balance.

It increases the responsibility for one's own health and stimulates the willingness to complete the projects and the interest is quickly lost, helping to develop constancy, consistency and to find the right motivations.

Being quick people in acquiring anything in the short term, they are overwhelmed by boredom and therefore leave the project alone.

A positive aspect of this essence is given by emotional balance, by self-confidence, by the ability to reach the goals by taking responsibility for one's own health without being distressed, while usually the people who need this essence lose a lot of time and energies, they are depressed in front of their own inconsistency and they feel frustrated in front of every loss.

People who easily lose the interest of an activity or project after they have started it.

They have difficulty stabilizing their emotions, since they always dominate changing and extreme moods. When they are in a bad mood they are aggressive and sharp with others.

- Monotonous, boring, without common sense, unwilling and fearful of diseases. They are afraid of old age, of pollution, of getting intoxicated or being infected if they visit a patient.

In general they dissipate their energy and time and this leads them to always lose opportunities, which is why they get depressed and frustrated.
The flower provides physical and mental stability.
It develops willpower to reach goals without apologizing for fear.
The dominant emotions in this flower are: frustration, depression, depression, lack of enthusiasm, boredom, fear of physical deterioration, inability to express and assimilate love or dominate hatred.

- Peach Flowered Tea Tree is a balancing of the pancreas also for insulin addictions.

The positive aspects of Peach Flowered Tea Tree are emotional balance, self-confidence, the ability to achieve goals, and to take responsibility for one's health, without excessive worries.

Bach flowers for the third chakra

Bach flowers - or Bach flower remedies - are an alternative medicine designed by the British physician Edward Bach, born on September 24, 1886 in Moseley by a Gallese family in England.

He graduated in medicine in 1912 and immediately worked in the emergency room of the university hospital where he began to get noticed for the large amount of time he dedicated to patients. He was immediately critical of other doctors, as they studied the disease as if it were separate from the individual, without focusing on the patients themselves. It is well known that our emotional states have a profound influence on our well-being and our health. An altered emotional state that repeats itself every day creates real dysfunctions of our body.

90% of the causes of human diseases come from plans that lie beyond the physical, and it is on these floors that the symptoms begin to manifest themselves before the physical body shows any disturbance. If we can identify the negative moods that come up when we get sick, we can fight the disease better and heal faster. Using floral remedies we try to influence the deeper structures from which the disease originates.

Bach Flowers rebalance emotions. They only address how we react emotionally to the vicissitudes, experiences and problems of our days. They give a great serenity and peace, courage or strength, they help us to feel in full of our possibilities.

They can be useful in the face of an illness, not from the physical point of view but just as a support for the mood. The person is seen as a complete individual where emotions are a pivotal point, and not just as a physical body with symptoms. It is therefore necessary to analyze the emotional state and not the physical symptoms, according to this the suitable remedies are found. In fact, subjects with identical physical problems react and live with different emotions and feelings. Bach flowers have no contraindications and do not interact with drugs.

Bach has thus divided the 38 flowers from which the remedies are taken. The very first flowers discovered by Bach were the so-called "12 Healers", which the Welsh doctor promptly began to experiment first on himself and then on his patients; the other 26 were discovered a short time later, divided into "7 Aids" and "19 Assistants".

Dr Bach later abandoned the distinction between "Healers", "Helpers" and "Assistants" considering it superfluous, but many people in the world continue to use it equally. Bach Flowers do not help to repress negative attitudes, but turn them into their positive side. Bach flowers associated with the second chakra are only for general reasons, because flowers are still chosen based on emotion that is not in harmony that should be balanced.

Cerato

It belongs to the category of "Healers".

Who needs this flower is a person who has little confidence in what he thinks, constantly asks advice to everyone, for every little thing. The person with this nature is really unbearable because he asks a thousand questions, for example when he is shopping he asks the cured meat what is the best product and his thought, this happens everywhere: from the hairdresser, to a seminar, to the university, to the specialist, and if he meets a person on the street he makes him the third degree.

Indecision is the key word of Cerato, although in reality it is a lack of trust in one's intuitions. The search for confirmation in others occurs due to a lack of trust in one's ability to grasp the essence of things.

When they find themselves having to make a decision, contrary to the Scleranthus type, they have no hesitation or difficulty in deciding. However, at a later stage, they start to have doubts and no longer feel so sure that they have made the right decision. So they start asking for opinions and advice from others and end up finding themselves totally confused. Cerato is the remedy to restore confidence in one's own judgment to people in this state of mind, so that they are able to listen to their own inner voice and to rely on their intuition.

Scleranthus

It belongs to the category of "Healers".

Who needs this flower is a person who can not make a decision between two things, when it seems that it is just one, then immediately thinks that the other is right.

This person is always undecided and is his inner torment, but he never talks about it with anyone. The mood changes easily passing quickly from happiness to sadness.

Faced with the need to choose between two options, one is in crisis trying to evaluate the pros and cons of each possibility with the risk of being bogged down in a dead end and with the risk of not trusting one's intuition.

Scleranthus is very useful in balance problems such as car and sea sickness.

With Scleranthus the balance and the clarity of one's choices are the basis of existence. The remedy is used to help the person to act with more decision and to understand what he really wants.

Impatiens

It belongs to the category of "Healers".

Who needs this flower is an impatient person, speaks, eats, dresses, works and walks quickly, thinks something and immediately acts. You do everything in a hurry, going from one thing to another.

Slow people are not tolerated, so much so that they prefer to be alone at their own pace, rather than behind the times of others. Impatiens people need to learn that speed is not equal to frenzy.

An additional symptom of Impatiens is the intractability as soon as you wake up.

With Impatiens you live your own and others rhythm with patience and availability. Impatiens concentrate is indicated for those who are easily irritable.

Because of the impatience felt, the person thinks he has to do everything right away, and for this he adopts a high speed in his actions, in his thoughts and even in his way of speaking. Their competence and efficiency cause them to be irritated and frustrated by slower colleagues and therefore prefer to work alone.

Because of her strong sense of independence she hates wasting time unnecessarily, and in conversations she often ends the sentences of others in their place.

Gentian

It belongs to the category of "Healers".

Who needs this flower is a pessimistic person, constantly considers the worst side of everything, sees the glass always half empty, his point of view is constantly negative even in the most banal situations, and in his projects he prepares each time to the negative in order not to be disappointed, so if the result has not been achieved, it can always be said that it was waiting for it. It is sad, depressed, every obstacle is knocked down and one is tempted to abandon. The cause of this sadness is generally known, there is a tendency to always have a sort of mistrust, even towards happiness. Gentian depression is always motivated by an objective or mental situation that momentarily holds back our goals. You do not feel down for no reason but you know what causes doubt or sadness. Gentian allows you to get up by evaluating new ways and new ways to achieve our goals.

With Gentian one has faith in what one feels, and in what happens in one's life. The person with this nature will change his way of seeing life, will not lose confidence at the first obstacle, pessimism will turn into optimism, it will be noticed above all in the eyes.

Gorse

It belongs to the "Aid" category. Who needs this flower is a person who lives a suffering that is prolonged in time, or unexpected. This state of mind is also born in those who are optimistic, because being a person who always manages to find the positive side of situations and therefore also adapt to what is unpleasant in life, comes to the conclusion that this is how they go things. You no longer have the strength to do anything about the problem you have, but then you still try something just because someone else pushes you to move.

The despair present in the locked state of Gorse stands out from other types of abatement because in this case has not yet taken hold and tries, even trying many ways, to get out of it.

Gorse increases confidence in their goals and in their destiny without letting go. With Gorse you have hope in your destiny. It is interesting to note that Gorse was entered by dr. Bach in the group of Remedies for uncertainty and not in that for despair, as in the case of Sweet Chestnut.

This shows that the main problem for people in the Gorse mood is the loss of certainty. Therefore, if you can persuade them to see things in a different light, trust and hope are renewed in them and they can begin to move forward with greater confidence. The Gorse Remedy helps to achieve all this.

It is interesting to note that Gorse was entered by dr. Bach in the group of Remedies for uncertainty and not in that for despair, as in the case of Sweet Chestnut. This shows that the main problem for people in the Gorse mood is the loss of certainty.

Therefore, if you can persuade them to see things in a different light, trust and hope are renewed in them and they can begin to move forward with greater confidence.

The Gorse Remedy helps to achieve all this.

Hornbeam

It belongs to the category of "Assistants".

Who needs this flower is a person who has a great difficulty getting out of bed in the morning, he wakes up already stressed as if he had just finished a run, a great job, and his need is to sleep, but more she is in bed and the more she gets tired.

Once you get off the bed, the person has a lot of difficulty getting dressed, washing, and as time passes, the energy magically returns; this happens because it begins to consume exciting substances like coffee, tea, cigarette, chocolate.

With Hornbeam every day is a new beginning and gives vitality and growth stimuli. You are mentally and physically fresh and lively. The floral remedy helps the person especially in the initial push and make it feel lighter and more elastic. The person will be able to complete his work without pauses due to exhaustion.

Wild Oat

It belongs to the "Aid" category.

Who needs this flower is a person who never finds satisfaction in everything he thinks or does. He always has a thousand ideas to put into action, many intuitions and at the end only indecisions, he decides continuously and also takes the initiative but while he is running he changes his mind, project or other. His dissatisfaction is evident in all its aspects.

Indecision is generalized, not between two things.

- When choosing from a multitude of possibilities is difficult, Wild Oat helps you take your own path. Classic example of the young person in front of the choice of the appropriate school when all or many of them seem suitable.

We would like to do something important but we do not know what. Wild Oat allows you to get in touch with your skills and your intuition.

The state of indecision of type Wild Oat is different from that of type Scleranthus, because in the second case the doubt is not about which direction to take, but rather about how to proceed or what to choose, while having clear the various alternatives.

- On the other hand, Wild Oat people do not know what the alternatives are because they have not yet defined their goals.

The remedy helps these people to understand their true role, making them rediscover their purpose in life, so that they can clearly understand which way to go. With Wild Oat you are able to do everything you like, even if the interests are multiple, you know your destination.

Crab Apple

It belongs to the category of "Assistants".

Who needs this flower is a person who believes not to be completely clean, as if he wanted to chase away some poison from his body, an evil that has now been generated, or that he thinks he has.It has the feeling of being dirty , polluted, both physically and psychologically.

Also suitable for all those who do not accept.

It is definitely the flower that has the greatest impact with the external shape, therefore with the skin and with our relationship with the body and the appearance. With Crab Apple it is easier to accept oneself for what you are, evaluating more our positive aspects without remaining anchored to the physical aspect alone. Useful even when obsessed with cleaning.

Given its relationship with the skin it becomes part of the Rescue Cream. The person with this character will accept more willingly; the floral remedy helps to alleviate phobias concerning dirt and contact with things that do not belong to your home environment such as going to public baths, fears that you can endanger your health and manage to stay in touch even with apparently unclean people. It can be applied in the form of cream on pimples, blisters, eczema, in short, any rash.

Vine

It belongs to the "Aid" category.

Who needs this flower is a person who wants to command everyone: he is a leader, a leader, a tyrant. In life he can not bear being commanded, but rather loves to command; he is always in charge of something, of a company, of a team, of a group, of the family, making decisions for everyone because he is in the certainty of doing their own good.

Leader and dictator, what a huge difference. These two figures are the positive and negative representation of Vine. In the blocked phase, Vine wants to convince others by dominating them, deciding for them.

Often Vine people have important roles in the work and in their interests and in the transformed state they can be excellent leaders by inciting and guiding others without obliging them and above all with respect for others.

They are very different from Vervain people who instead try to convert others to their own way of thinking, instead the Vine types impose orders and discipline without admitting replies.

The remedy develops this positive side of the Vine personality. With Vine, one's authority is lived with trust in oneself and in others. It is also known to delegate to others, thus evaluating also the potential of others.

Number of the third chakra

In the third chakra there are ten petals which, when they turn, can appear as a vortex.

- Ten brings with it a great charge of esoteric meaning that is made evident by the fact that a pregnancy lasts for ten lunar months, in many versions of the Kabbalah there are ten sephirot, the most used numerical system in the world is the decimal one.

People have ten fingers they use to count, leading to an innate adoption of the Ten as a basis in the intuitive numerical system. It should be noted that Dieci is considered a modern completion number because it is only in the last few centuries that it has been used as a basic block of numerical systems, currency and measurement. When Ten replaced the Twelve as the supreme number, it brought about a change in human mental patterns by making them more scientific in the approach to esoteric matters (Twelve's supporters disagree with this last statement). The fate indicated by the Ten linked to the date of birth must always be compared to the number One and indicates:

- To the positive - creative and artistic life, individuality and a lot of pride. The subject will be inclined to loneliness and to work alone, inevitably achieving success.

- To the negative - who has this number by sum, will have to try to overcome selfishness and vanity.

The Ten was sacred to the Pythagoreans, who loved to represent it through the Tetratkys (a sort of equilateral triangle composed of 10 points: the base of 4, then to rise 3, 2, 1).

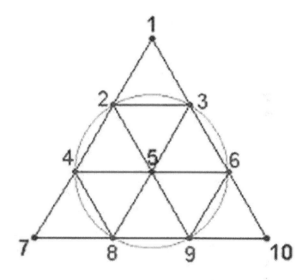

For the Pythagoreans ten were also the celestial entities: Sun, Moon, Earth, the five planets visible to the naked eye: Mercury, Venus, Mars, Jupiter and Saturn, the Sky of the fixed stars plus the Antiterra, an invisible planet because in opposition to the Earth compared to the sun.

- The numbers Ten will therefore be ambitious, cerebral, but selfish and will succeed in business even if they must possess great willpower to overcome the obstacles they will encounter on their journey. They may be envious of their friends and feel the tendency to annihilate their competitors without mercy. They will certainly be solitary and may even become enlightened heads of state, but also despots and tyrants.

The number Ten symbolizes perfection, as well as the annulment of all things.

- $10 = 1 + 0 = 1$ illustrates the eternal start over.

The Ten is the total of the first four numbers and therefore contains the globality of the universal principles. Corresponds, as already said, to the Pythagorean Tetraktys, which together with the seven considered it the most important number, as it is formed by the sum of the first four digits ($1 + 2 + 3 + 4 = 10$), expresses the totality, the fulfillment, the final realization.

- The Tetraktys represented the number 10 and was drawn as a triangle made of points: four on each side, a point in the middle (or, a point on the highest level, two immediately below, then three, and finally four).

The figure is a geometric arrangement that expresses a number or, if desired, a number expressed through a geometric arrangement. The concept that it presupposes is that of the measurable order. Esoterically, the vertex of the triangle, the highest point, is the Logos; the complete triangle is the Tetrade or Triangle in the Square, which is the double symbol of the four-letter Tetragrammaton in the manifested Cosmos, and of its triple root radius (its Noumenon) in the unmanifest.

- Pythagoras, as is known, associated the point at 1, the line at 2, the surface at 3, the solid at 4; these values are easily found by looking at the figure from top to bottom.

The sides that close the points of the Tetrade represent the barriers of matter, or noumenic substance, and separate the triangle from the world of thought. For Pythagoras, the Triangle was the first conception of manifested Divinity, its image, Father-Mother-Son; the Quaternary, on the other hand, was the perfect number, the ideal, noumenical root of all numbers and things on the physical plane. The number Ten is divine because perfect, in that it brings together in a new unity all the principles expressed in the numbers one to nine. For this reason the number Ten is also called Heaven, to indicate both the perfection and the dissolution of all things, for the fact that it contains all the possible numerical relations.

Phisical exercises

Exercise 1

Do some relaxation exercise by shaking your arms and legs.
Sit on the floor with your back upright and then perform alternate breathing for a few minutes.

Exercise 2

Assume the position of the quadruped and perform the "horse's back / arched back of the cat" exercise 7 times.

Exercise 3

Sit with legs closed and stretched forward straight and resting on the ground.
Put your palms on the ground next to the buttocks, with the fingers pointing backwards.
Inhaling, bring the basin upwards; in this way, the whole bust should form a line with the rest of the body.
Replace the pelvis when you exhale.
Repeat the exercise 3 times.

Exercise 4

Put your hands in front of your chest while sitting.
The right thumb over the left thumb, both positioned between the palms, while the other fingers, facing upwards, encircle the thumbs, on which you can exert light pressure.
Close the eyes, inhale deeply through the nose and exhale repeatedly pronounced the mantra "ram".
Repeat 7 times by focusing on the navel.

Exercise 5

Lie down on your back and close your eyes.
Leave behind all the worries of everyday life and observe your inner life (thoughts, emotions, body).
Then place your hands above your navel on your stomach and stomach.
Let the breath flow when you inhale and exhale, imagining that you will receive energy from the cosmos, which will flow into your solar plexus, seeing this energy of a beautiful yellow color with your mind.
Repeat for 5 minutes, then lay your hands on the ground and relax.

Recommended stones for the 3rd Chakra

In crystallotherapy, stones of the 3rd Chakra are considered to be those of yellow color, of any type of gloss or transparency.

The crystals that can rebalance the third chakra are amber, yellow chalcedony, yellow calcite, sun stone, tiger's eye, pyrite, citrine quartz, rutilated quartz, imperial topaz.

The area of placement of the stones is just above the navel.

Feel the energy that passes through the sacral chakra while you hold it in your hand or carry it through a ring or necklace. You do not have to buy them all, just choose the stones you prefer or which you already own.

Amber

The word Amber comes from the Arabic Anbar, which initially indicated a waxy substance produced by the sperm of the Sperm whale. Obviously, the Amber we know does not refer to that type of product, but to a mixture of fossilized organic compounds (resin).

The first resin produced by trees, ancestors of the current conifers, dates back to about 250 million years ago, that is during the Mesozoic period. But how did the process of fossilization that led to the creation of this extraordinary gift of nature, improperly called stone?

- The resin, produced by very large trees, was deposited on the soil starting the first phase of fossilization called polymerization. The next process, called precisely fossilization, occurs after about 5 million years giving the result that glassy substance, called Amber.

The amber, to be defined as such, must be at least 150,000 years, otherwise it is Copale or Copalite which are organic resins that are not old enough (less than 100,000 years) and not yet fossilized and hard enough to become amber. Amber has always been considered a strongly protective and anti-demonic amulet. Highly protective, it also helps in the manifestation of one's ideas in everyday reality.

It strengthens the solar plexus, gives mental clarity, balance and confidence in its possibilities.

- Amber can help metabolic deficiencies, hearing problems and stomach upset. In Poland, amber tincture is still considered an effective remedy for cold, throat and respiratory tract problems. Amber powder is inhaled to bring relief to respiratory problems.

The life force within amber promotes fertility and its protective and environmental compensatory properties make it a remedy to be used to prepare for healing or motherhood. Amber gives light energy that is soothing and energizing at the same time. Regenerate the environment by pulling out heavy negativity, if burned. Remember to always clean and purify amber if used for crystal therapy and never leave amber in the sun as it can become fragile. Amber is excellent if accompanied by jaietto, fossil jasper and carnelian.

- Amber has the power to transmute negative energies into positive energies. But, beyond this great faculty, it is used as a calming of the whole nervous system.

Amber also amplifies its intellectual predispositions and abilities. In general it is thought that this "stone" can act on our whole body purifying our energies, giving us a deep sense of warmth. This means that our body is always protected from possible illness.

The Chakra associated with it is the 3rd, that of the Navel and the Solar Plexus, while its zodiacal sign is Leo.

Yellow calcite

Calcite owes its name to the Latin word "calx" which means "lime", because for calcite the main component is limestone.

There is a deep link between the yellow calcite stone and that of the animal and plant kingdoms and in all of nature; the real ability to move forward in spite of external influences by taking an active part in what we are creating in our lives.

- The yellow calcite stone is very known for its propensity to purification, cleanliness and in harmony with the regenerating and revitalizing power of nature itself. Yellow calcite is used to remove the old patterns (blocks) of the old stagnant energy present in us and to increase personal motivation and sense of unity.

It is an excellent stone for the study of the arts and sciences and to amplify and increase any type of energy, thanks to the double refraction property discovered in stone in 1669 by Erasmo Bartholinus. Yellow calcite can help bones and joints and balances the amount of calcium in the body, helping to improve the absorption of important vitamins and minerals in the body.

The properties of yellow calcite are a good help for remote energy work, given the power of amplification that can be sent.

- This property, together with fluorescence, phosphorescence, and thermoluminescence, have allowed since ancient times to use yellow calcite in spells and ritual magic.

Eye of the Tiger

The stone called "tiger's eye" is a quartz crystal, with beautiful bands of golden yellow that cross it. It is a powerful mineral that helps harmony and balance, improving states of anxiety and fear.

- Stimulates action and helps make decisions with discernment and understanding, as well as with great mental clarity. Traditionally it is used as an amulet against negative energies, and is known to induce courage, self-confidence and willpower. It enhances creativity and is one of the stones that help the awakening of Kundalini.

Of the tiger eye stone it is known the reputation of marvelous gem to attract material wealth (and to improve the stability necessary to maintain such wealth), abundance, stimulate the growth of Kundalini energy and therefore personal vitality. Most of these stones come from South Africa, but are also found in Brazil, India, Burma, Australia and the United States.

- The meaning of the name "tiger's eye" derives from the fact that it resembles the feline iris: the color goes from yellow to brown and brown, crossed by beautiful striped nuances.

The mineral is a great energy amplifier, as in most cases of quartz crystals, and will in turn increase the energy of all the other crystals with which it is used.

The particular movement, almost liquid, of the light that reflects through the stone itself, has always made the tiger's eye an excellent tool for the vision or for the works of divination. The stone combines the energy of the Earth with that of the Sun, keeping strong the rooting of the person who uses it, thus revealing an excellent meditation stone. Improve your courage and tenacity, allowing these attributes to always be balanced with mental clarity and a joyful vision.

- The properties of the tiger's eye are also used to discern the truth in every situation and to help understand the life you are living.

The benefits can help slow the flow of energy through the body, which makes the gem very useful for stress-related illnesses.

Excellent stone for arthritis and inflammation of the bone tissue. It is said to be useful in cases of schizophrenia, various mental disorders and impulsive obsession. It promotes the best energy flow through the body when worn, making it an excellent stone for concentration, especially for those with attention deficits.

- This stone vibrates a lot with the sacral chakra (or navel) and gives a useful energy to improve creativity.

Its vibration within this chakra also helps distracted or listless people to take on commitments and carry them out, as it gives courage and fortitude. The golden stones, in general, help to strengthen the male principle: the fire, or the solar element in this crystal, stimulates the ability to manifest the most ardent desires. Because the tiger's eye binds to the ground through the basic chakra, it helps to be calmer and centered: in other words, it allows you to take the necessary steps to be more practical in life. With the tiger's eye, the Kundalini energy increase is also stimulated, the coiled snake that resides at the base of the vertebral column. When stimulated, it can rise through the spine: it is said that this process can lead to enlightenment.

If you want to use the tiger's eye for this purpose, you can combine with it the serpentine, which in turn will facilitate the process of awakening of the Kundalini.

- It is suggested to use the tiger's eye in combination with hyaline quartz, serpentine and the Moonstone.

Pyrite

Pyrite, owes its term from the Greek "pyros" literally "fire", given the formation of sparks when it is hit.

The French call the pyrite "Pierre de Santé", which means "stone of health", given the strong conviction already before the Middle Ages of its positive effects on health in general.

Pyrite, due to its resemblance to gold, has made it a strong traditional symbol in all latitudes and cultures in the world to attract money and good luck. Moreover, the pyrite symbolizes the warmth and the vital and lasting presence of the sun, favoring the recall of beautiful memories of love and friendship.

- Pyrite can help by giving a feeling of greater vitality during periods of hard work or stress.

Pyrite can increase physical endurance, stimulate the intellect and help transform thought into intelligent action. Strongly recommended for people who face great conceptual ideas daily, in the business, arts or education world. Its properties strengthen mental abilities and awareness of higher forms of knowledge. It can improve communication skills by removing anxiety and frustration. Creative and intuitive impulses can be more stimulated if used together with fluorite and calcite.

Stone of the Sun.

The sunstone is also known as heliolite, whose meaning derives from the Greek "helios" which means "sun" and "lithos" meaning "stone". The sun stone was used in ancient Greece to represent the Sun God, Helios (or Apollo). In Greece it was believed that the sunstone invigorated and improved the state of the physical body and the spirit, bringing renewed health to both. This particular gem was appreciated by the ancient magicians, who used the stone of the sun to attract the power of the sun by associating it with power and material wealth. The properties of the sunstone are known for its powerful connection to light and the power of the sun, giving it a sunny character. It brings light to all situations, and is an optimal stone for the solar plexus chakra.

- It is a powerful stone to dispel fears and phobias of all kinds, increases will, as well as personal vital energy. It can provide the resilience and energy needed to undertake projects and activities that can find objective obstacles.

Excellent for chronic sore throat and to alleviate the pain of gastric ulcers.
Also used for cartilage, rheumatism and general pains. It also helps to find and maintain a fruitful sexual relationship. Reached closely, it stimulates the personal power of attraction.

The property of the sunstone is enhanced if used together with the moonstone, especially in solstices, in personal rituals, in energy works and spells. Together they represent the balance of power between physical characteristics and psychic and spiritual characteristics.

The stone of the sun is very useful in removing energy bonds or karmic wires from other people or things, and turns out to be a fundamental stone in crystal therapy given the increase in energy that can be added to other stones.

Citrine quartz

The citrine quartz stone is named after citrin, an old French word meaning yellow.

Almost all the citrine that is available on the market today is actually the amethyst stone (the one with the lowest value and beauty) that is subjected to a high heat treatment. The natural citrine quartz goes from a pale yellow to a more intense yellow. All that is dark orange, brown, until reddish brown, has been heat treated. The only exception to this is the darker citrine named Citrino Madeira, named for the similarity of color to Madeira wines.

It is a stone that in ancient times was used as a protection against poisons and psychic disorders.

Citrine quartz increases the healing energy of the physical body and opens the conscious mind to intuition. An energizing crystal, invigorating against chronic and highly beneficial fatigue, also increases internal motivation and promotes physical activity, which in turn improves digestion and helps the cleaning organs.

It can also work as a detoxifier for the blood. It develops inner calm and security and makes us less sensitive and more open to constructive criticism. It can dispel negative feelings and helps us to accept the flow of events. Citrine quartz can eliminate self-defeating behaviors or such tendencies and increase self-esteem.

- It is also known as a "success" stone because it is able to promote personal success and abundance, especially in business and commerce.

Citrine quartz can increase one's optimism in every situation, bringing a more positive vision into the subconscious mind, allowing one to enter the flow of things with better results. Highly protective, it can be easily programmed for your personal protection, this makes it an excellent tool for transmuting negative energy.
It can help memory, willpower and motivate greater self-discipline.

Rutilated quartz

Rutilated quartz is a type of quartz which has an ageless shape inside the rutile (titanium dioxide). The needles of rutile may be reddish, or may be of gold, of silver, or on very rare occasions, of a greenish color.

The inclusions of rutilated quartz are called since the Middle Ages, hair of Venus, and from that period comes the belief that the stone can slow down the aging process. Rutilated quartz is a stone that has both the energy of the energetic vibration of hyaline quartz, and the power of amplification of rutile, which makes it very useful when combined with other stones, especially labradorite, citrine quartz and chalcopyrite.

- The properties of rutilated quartz make it an illuminator for the soul, a stone to promote spiritual growth. The stone is known to be an energizing stone that helps in obtaining and releasing energy at all levels.

It is said that it can also alleviate the imposed loneliness and alleviate the feelings of guilt generated by others, thus making happiness possible.

It can increase its autonomy and self-esteem by infusing the ability to find its own way.

It is a useful stone for eating disorders, and the absorption of nutrients from food, tissue regeneration, fatigue, and depression. It is used for meditation, in spiritual communications, and work on lucid dreams.

A particularly suitable stone for the search for more spiritual experiences and meditation on feminine energies.

Rutilated quartz may be useful for moving energy along the meridians and in physical areas where energy stagnates.

Imperial Topaz

The golden-yellow topaz, as already mentioned, is called "imperial".
For the Hindu community, wearing this mineral close to the heart gives long life, beauty and intelligence.

- The ancient Egyptians believed that the yellow topaz protected from all negativity, associating the yellow color with the sun god Ra.
- In the same way, the Romans always connected the mineral to the sun.
- The ancient Greeks used it when they needed to restore their strength and to guarantee protection: they were in fact convinced they could approach the deities.

It is believed that the crystal is extremely energizing, being a hot stone. It promotes creativity, and brings a sense of trust and protection. Free from stale and negative energy, from fatigue and tension.
Some believe that imperial topaz, finally, is useful for preventing thefts and fires.
Last but not least, it would be effective in cases of insomnia, depression and panic attacks, as it gives a positive and optimistic attitude.

Finally, it strengthens the flow of energy, protects the heart, improves blood circulation, relieves pain from rheumatoid arthritis, protects kidneys, liver and endocrine glands.

Printed in Great Britain
by Amazon